I WANT MY BODY BACK

A GUIDE TO YOUR BEST BODY: FOR MEN, WOMEN, AND FAMILIES

Lillie Franks

AUTHOR. COACH. SPEAKER. MENTOR

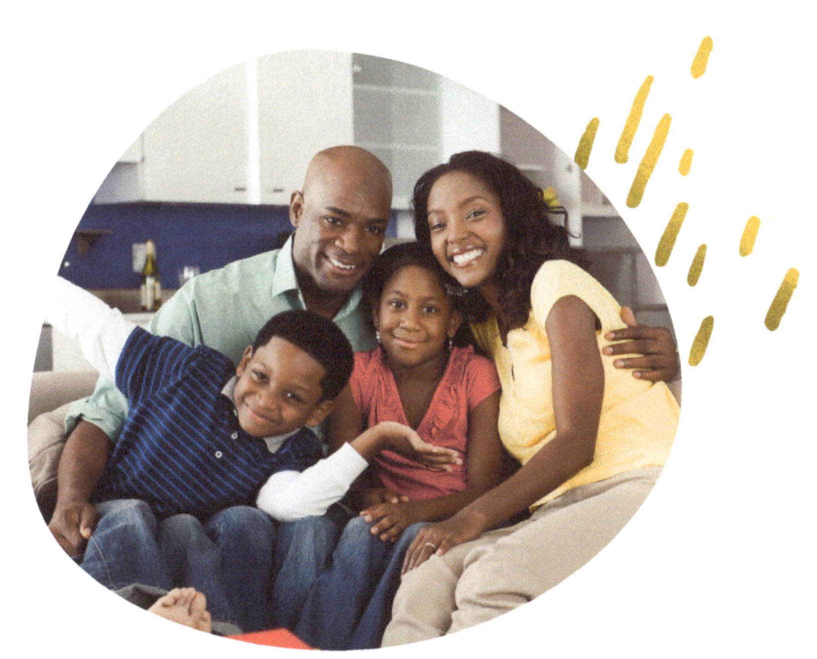

CONTENTS

FOREWORD

WELCOME

THANK YOU!

ARISE!

WHAT'S GOING ON WITH ME?

CONSULT WITH YOUR PHYSICIAN

BAD EATING HABITS

FIND GOD'S HEALING IN HIS WORD

START CREATING A NEW YOU

FINDING THE RIGHT BALANCE

DID YOU KNOW?

DO NOT FORGET, YOU ARE AWESOME

EAT FOR LIFE

FIND HEALING IN GOD'S WORD

LORD, GIVE ME STRENGTH IN MY PRAYER LIFE

SPEAK WHAT YOU WANT TO SEE

AFFIRMATIONS

WHAT DOES GOD SAY ABOUT STRESS?

LORD, I AM STRESSED OUT!

STRESS

START YOUR OWN RESEARCH ON DEVELOPING A HEALTHIER LIFE

IS YOUR LIFE GOING IN A CIRCLE?

GOD'S WORD CAN HEAL YOUR MIND

MINDSET

MY HEALTH MATTERS

FIND OUT WHAT'S WRONG, AND ASK GOD

WHAT YOU WILL NEED TO START

ENGAGE

HOW IS GOD TELLING YOU TO GET IN SHAPE

GETTING RESULTS

WHAT THE WORD OF GOD SAYS ABOUT HEALING LEAVES

10 TEAS WITH HEALING BENEFITS

A WINNER'S ATTITUDE

I'M GOING TO GET MY BODY BACK

IT'S ALL IN THE MIND

HOW TO REVERSE THE CURSE

WHAT'S EATING YOU?

I FEEL MUCH BETTER NOW!

5 WEEKS OF PERSONAL, MAJOR ACCOMPLISHMENTS

CERTIFICATE OF COMPLETION

REFERENCES & PUBLISHING INFO

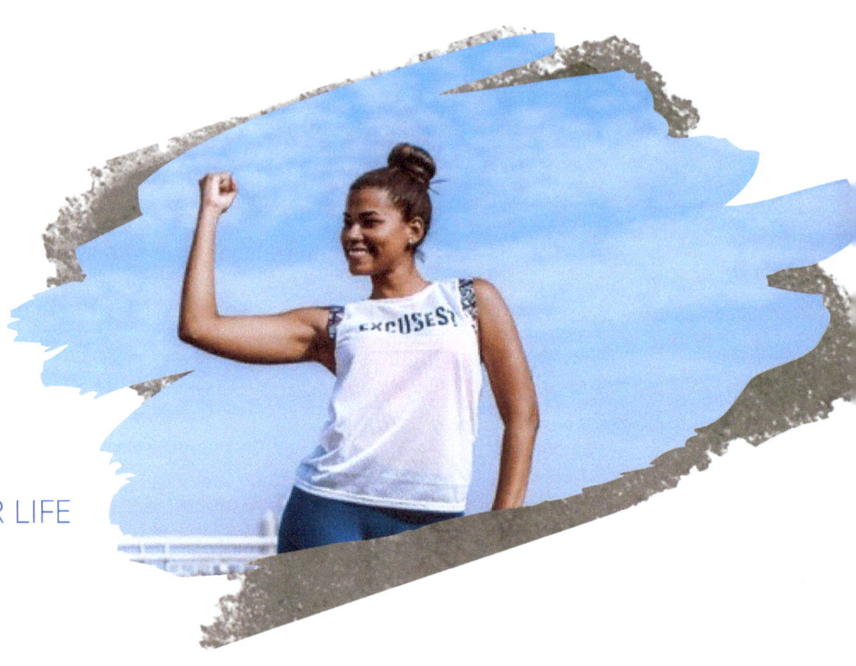

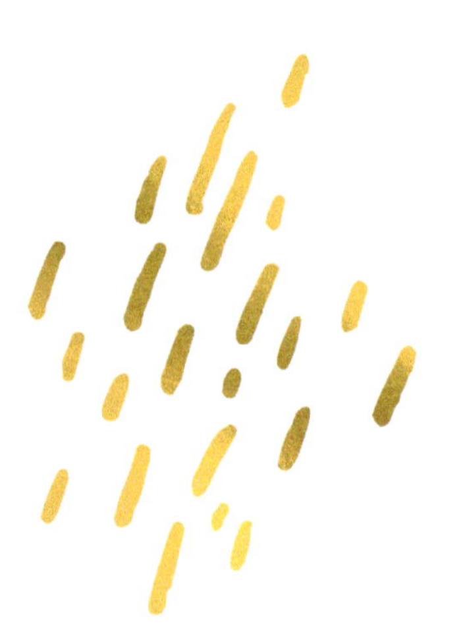

FOREWORD

I too was struggling to get my body back, until one day I was blessed to spend time with Coach Lillie; and in one conversation, my attitude about health changed. I had always been on the thin side and mostly healthy. As I began to grow older, I did not really take the time to take care of my health and my body. Consequently, I gained unwanted weight and my health began to fail. Like most, I did not know what to do. I made excuses, swept it under the rug, and ignored it until one day it hit me in the face like a ton of bricks. Coach Lillie came along at the right time--just when I decided I wanted my body back. She shared her testimony, some helpful tips, and an eating guide that I followed. Praise be to God! I am healthier and I have a physical manifestation of how her coaching plan and information can be beneficial and yield optimal results.

Merneen Spearman

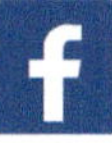

WELCOME

Come on and get your body back with Coach Lillie. I have used these strategies in this book to change my life, and I want to help you change yours for the better too. I turned my life around by not allowing sickness or injuries to make me feel defeated. You can feel the same. You can develop a workout plan using this easy-to-use Fitness Tracker for your mind, body, and spirit. As you get in touch with the "new you" you want to create, you will begin to grow spiritually and physically while improving your daily living. This book will guide you to feeling good and looking better. You will be able to chart your progress through interactive questions, meditation, and journal sheets.

You can declare, " I AM GETTING MY BODY BACK."

We focus on Meditation, the Word, and Worship. We will visit eating habits, drinking healthy, and we will focus on having a positive attitude for your new journey. Be refreshed as you concentrate on losing bad habits that keep you from becoming victorious. Become the person that you have the craving to be. Work hard and get the best result by telling yourself, "I Want My Body Back."

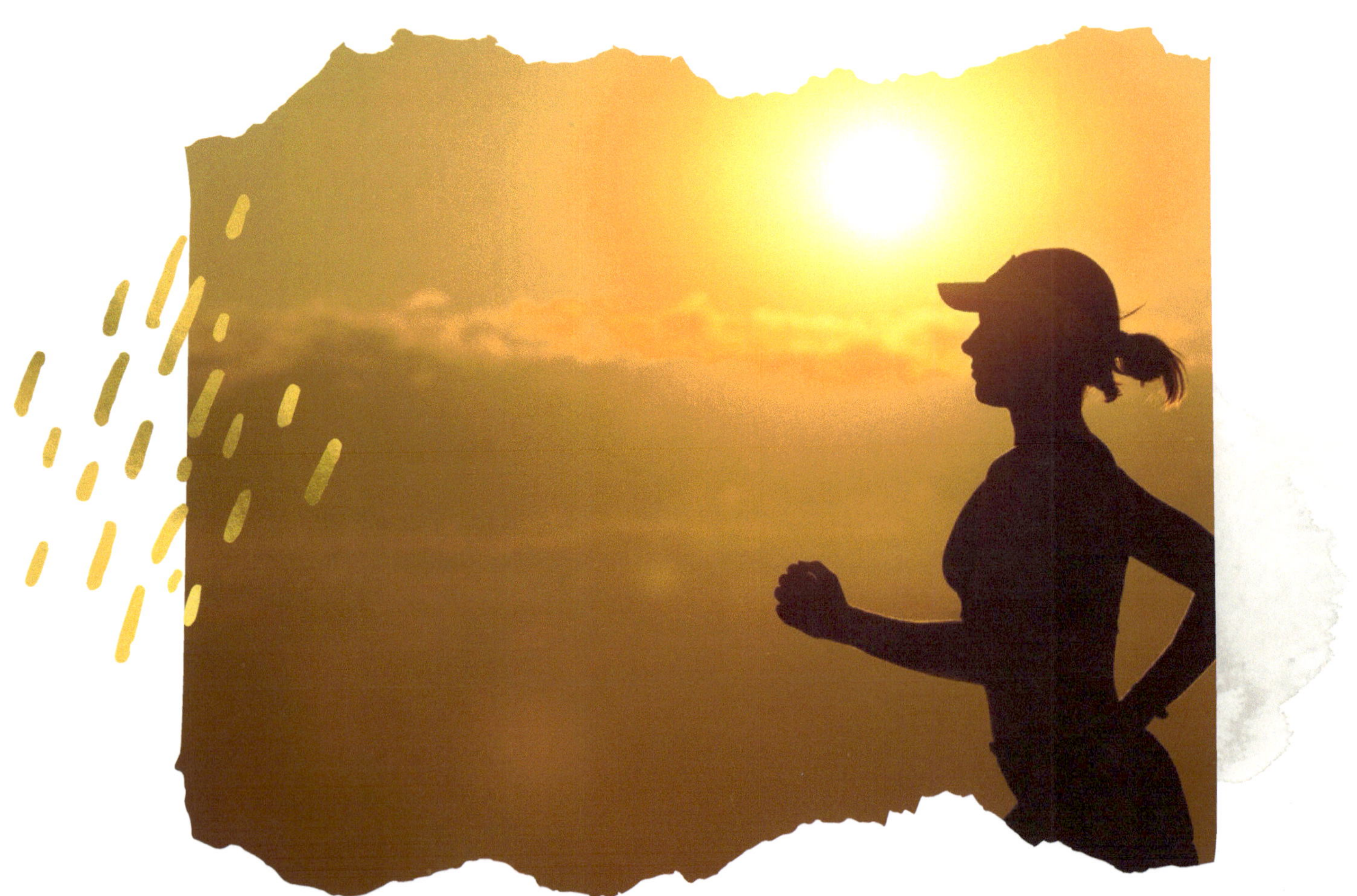

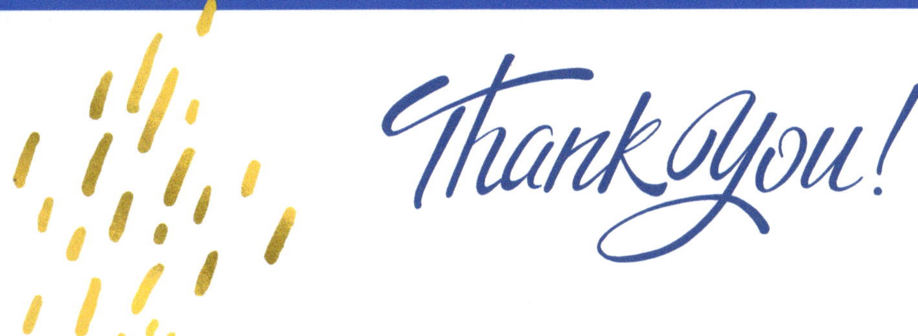

To my King - Michael Franks

I must say "thank you" for your love and support. You are my teammate4life. God has His hands all over your life, and you are a phenomenal man. I genuinely believe I can accomplish anything by being by your side. You are my king. I cannot thank you enough for all that you do for us. You are my heart, and you have all my love.

Lady Merneen - Lady M Publishing Company

My little sister. I appreciate you. You have always been a woman I admired, loved, and cherished from the time we met. We've been friends for over 39 years. Thank you for the laughter, the worship, and the wisdom you shared while collaborating on this book's design. You did a beautiful job! You have a spirit of excellence in all that you do. You are amazing. We are sisters indeed, born to encourage each other to grow stronger together. I love you, and I always will. We did it, and "I thank you!"

Venita Govan, PhD

We were destined to be friends. Our paths crossed so many times in the halls of McClure North High School, but it wasn't time for us to take the journey of life then, but it is now! Thank you for your love and support and for editing my first book, "Sisters In My Village," and I Want My Body Back. I appreciate you dearly. I praise God for our friendship, collaboration, and partnership. God always sends you to me whenever I am ready to release my thoughts to the world. Thank you for being a wonderful friend to me.

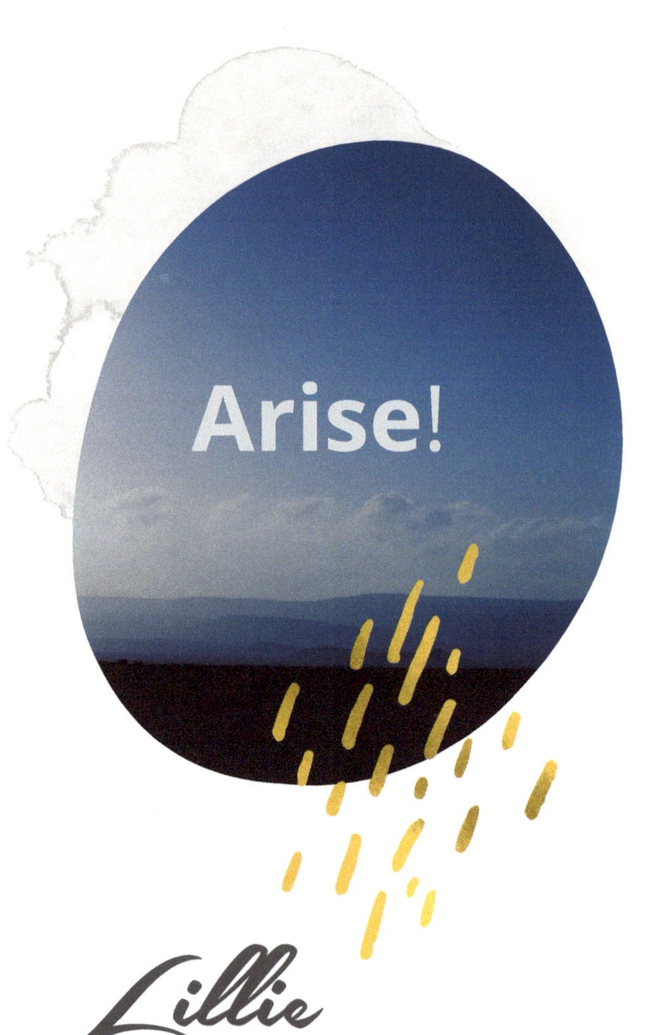

LET ME TELL YOU WHAT HAPPENED TO ME...

I have always been an active woman. I understand how my body works and what makes it feel great. Going for long walks and working out makes me feel good on the inside. But, there was a season when I wasn't working out at all. Work was overwhelming, and my home life was challenging within itself, and saying the least, I had nothing to give anyone. I was exhausted. I felt horrible. I felt like I was holding on to threads.

I kept telling myself that I was going to be all right. But, I was overwhelmed, and it seemed as if nothing would get better. Have you ever felt like everything was falling apart, including you? Think about it, and write down a short testimony about that moment.

Your Testimony:

Remember, no matter how bad you feel, you are in control of your health. If you don't feel like yourself, get a check-up. The statement that High Blood Pressure is a silent killer is true, but you have the power to get it under control. Every disease has symptoms; so, get help before it's too late. Study your body.

WHAT'S GOING ON WITH ME?

These things affect your body: High Blood Pressure, Decreased Stamina, Sugar Diabetes, Insomnia, Fatigue, Anxiety and Stress.

Write down precisely what is going on with you:

High blood pressure may go undetected.
Some of the affects of High Blood Pressure are:
·Severe headaches
·Severe anxiety
·Shortness of breath
·Spotty vision
·Pulsations in the neck or head

Do you have High Blood pressure? Y or N
Do you have some of these symptoms? Y or N
If so, please do what is necessary to get
your blood pressure under control.

Consult With Your Physician!

The information and suggestions in this book are for guidance, ideas, encouragement, and support. These steps and reflection were beneficial for my journey. Though our journeys are different, our ultimate goal is the same. Please consult with your physician while improving your health. Some of the techniques that were helpful for me may need to be revised for you to Get Your Body Back! Remember, consult with your physician!

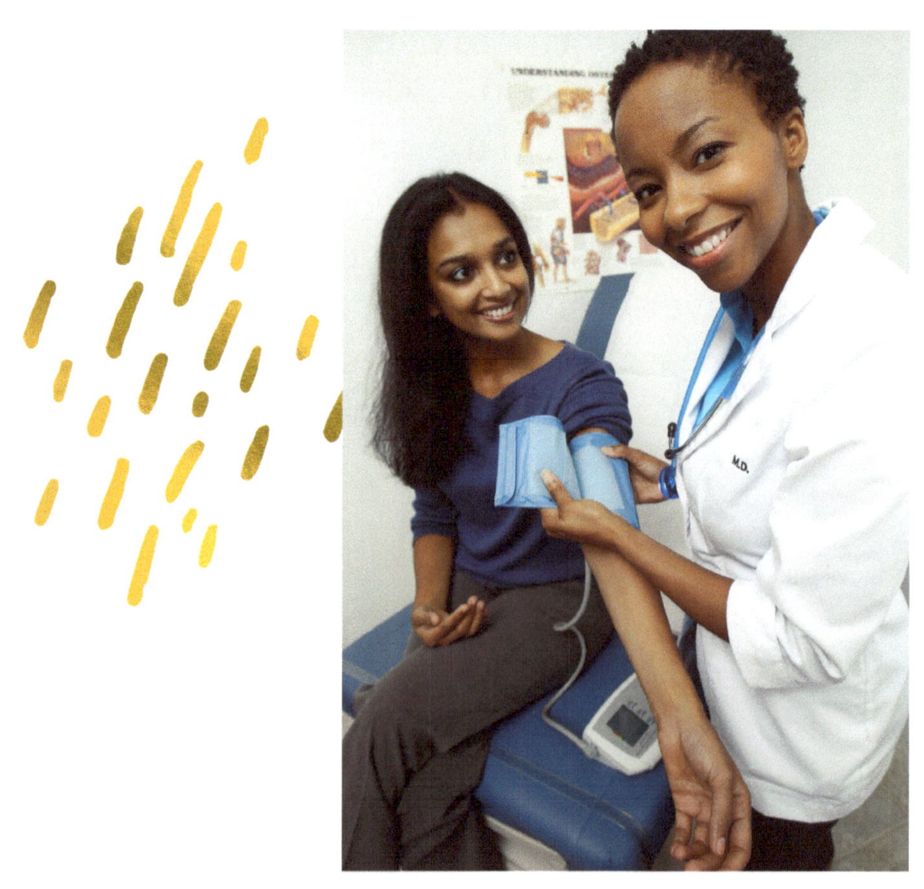

BAD EATING HABITS

Bad eating habits contribute to poor health and have harmful effects on the body. Check out your eating habits. Let's talk about your diet. What do you eat for breakfast? What do you eat for lunch? Do you plan what you are eating, or do you eat whatever comes to mind? I love fried foods. Yummy! I don't mean to make you hungry; but, hamburgers, french fries, chips, fried chicken, and baked potatoes (fully loaded) were my favorite meals when I needed something quick. My body craved all the wrong foods daily. After a while, my temple of God was in distress. I realized that I created this world all by myself.

I thought I was going to have a heart attack. My body changed, and I was no longer feeling great anymore. I made a doctor's appointment and found out that I had diabetes. I was devastated. My blood sugar level was horrible. I felt like I would die, but I wasn't ready. I wanted to live. I started researching this dreadful disease that was attacking my body. I decided **No More Tears,** it's time to do something.

I started educating myself about the effects this disease had on me. I found some shocking news that I would like to share with you.

My mother-in-law would always say, "When you know better, you ought to do better."

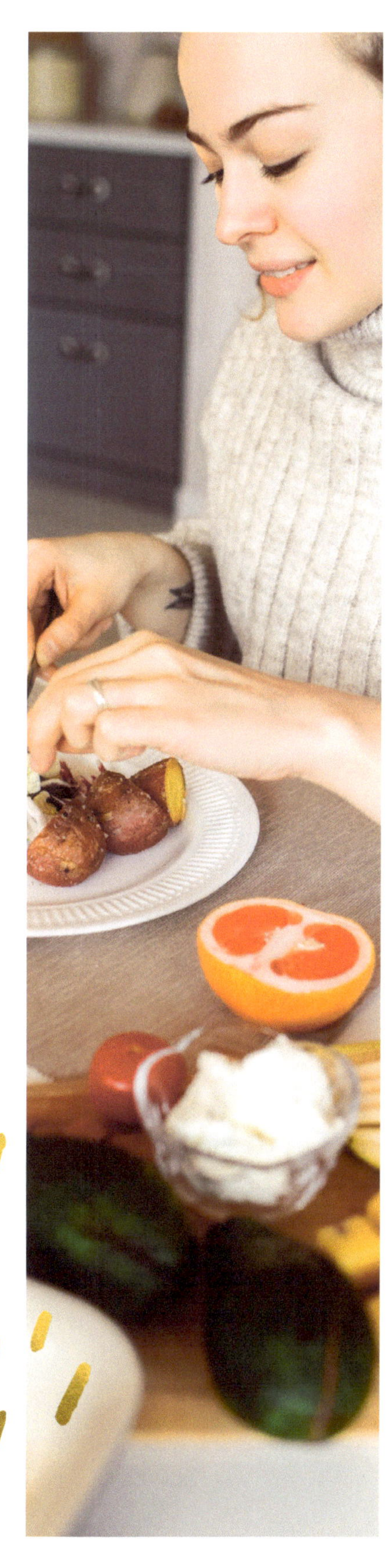

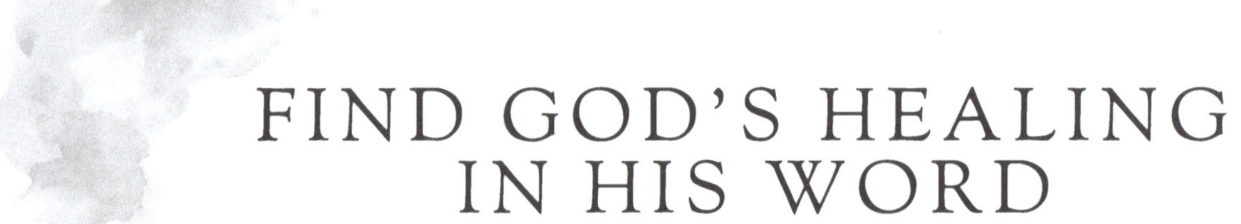

FIND GOD'S HEALING
IN HIS WORD

Everything that we need for our bodies has been created by God Almighty.

Exodus 23:25

"Worship the LORD your God, and his blessing will be on your food and water. I will take away sickness from among you..."

Jeremiah 17:14

"Heal me, O Lord, and I will be healed; save me and I will be saved, for you are the one I praise."

Exodus 15:26

He said, "If you listen carefully to the LORD your God and do what is right in his eyes, if you pay attention to his commands and keep all his decrees, I will not bring on you any of the diseases I brought on the Egyptians, for I am the LORD, who heals you."

James 5:14-15

"Is anyone among you sick? Let them call the elders of the church to pray over them and anoint them with oil in the name of the Lord. And the prayer offered in faith will make the sick person well; the Lord will raise them up. If they have sinned, they will be forgiven."

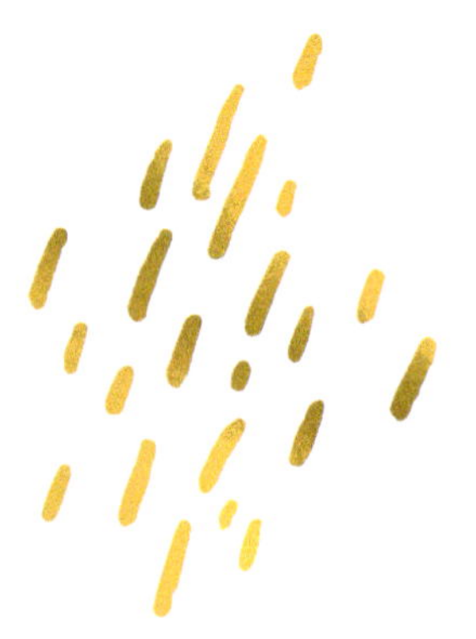

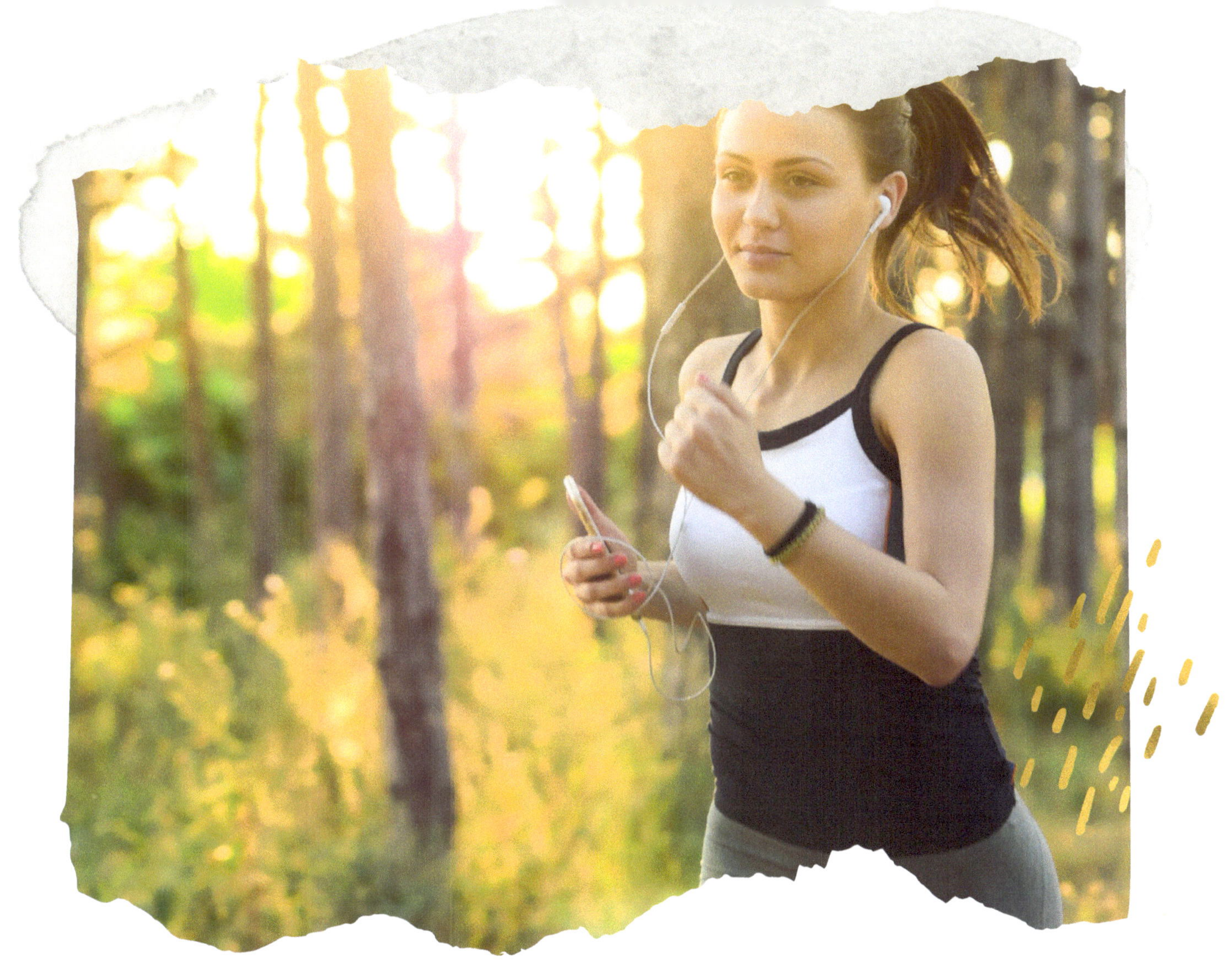

Start creating a new you.

Visualize what you need to do to start your new journey.
Think about exercise, what you are eating, your habits, your health issues, where you would like to see yourself health-wise in the next 21 days, and write what you visualize here:

____

____

____

____

____

____

____

FINDING THE RIGHT BALANCE

Start your morning off right. Drink one cup of warm lemon water or a cup of hot lemon tea. Lemon water will give you the vitamins that your body needs and may boost your immune system. Implement practices that will help build your immune system during this pandemic season. Make sure you take your vitamins daily. Think about it: What are you eating?

____

____

____

____

____

____

Ask yourself:

1. Am I eating to live or do I live to eat?
2. Do I completely understand the benefits of food?
3. Have I found the right balance for my life and body?

It's best to eat "Clean" food. "Clean" food means food in its whole form, or close to its complete form, that has been minimally refined or processed. So eating organic, clean food is the best food you can put into your body. Begin eating fresh foods that consist of lean meats, good carbs, and don't forget to load up on lots of vegetables, fruit, salad, and good fats. "Clean" food encourages you to consume more whole foods such as fruits, vegetables, lean proteins, whole grains, and healthy fats — and limits highly processed snack foods, sweets, and other packaged foods. Learn more about how to eat "clean." It's easier to digest "Clean" food because it's more efficient for your metabolism. "Clean" food helps you to receive the proper essentials, helping your to body work as a mean machine.

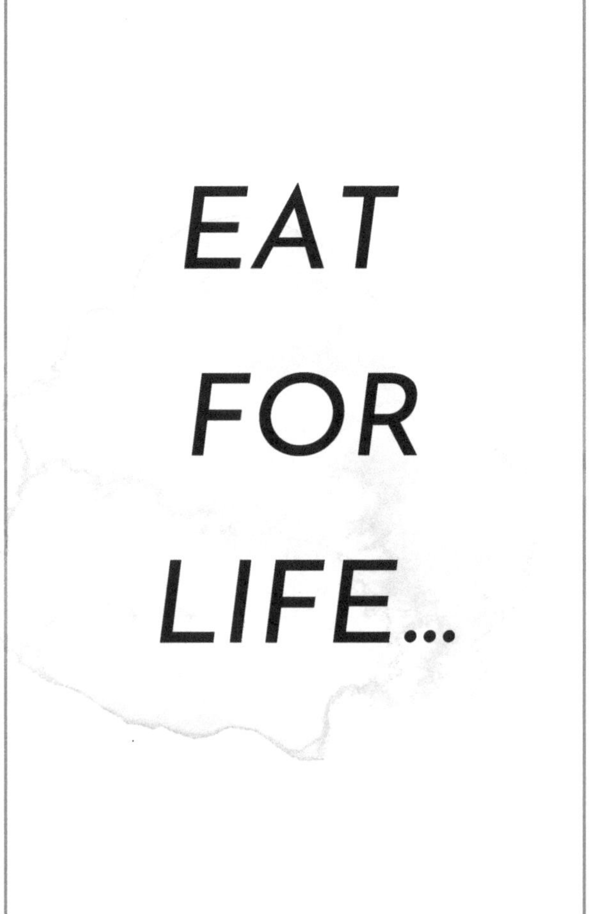

FINDING THE RIGHT BALANCE

Think about the things in your life that are stressing you out and the things you need to do when you are stressed out. Get fit and healthy. Exercise is refreshing and great for reducing stress. I use a combination of strength training, cardio, and meditation. Cardio keeps you fit and stops weight gain, and strength training shapes the body and makes you feel great. There are so many essential things that will help manage stress in your life. I workout several ways and do routines that take away stress and help me stay positive.

1. Go for a bike ride. I used to ride my bike for hours, but now I am limited because of a terrible accident, but I still go as long as I can. It's refreshing.
2. Put your tennis shoes on and go for a walk.
3. Take a nap. Even during lunchtime, find somewhere safe and take a rest on your lunch break.
4. Have a cup of tea and read a good book.
5. Join a gym.
6. Put on some music and dance until you feel the stress fall right off of you.
7. Read your Bible.
8. Call a friend and ask for prayer.

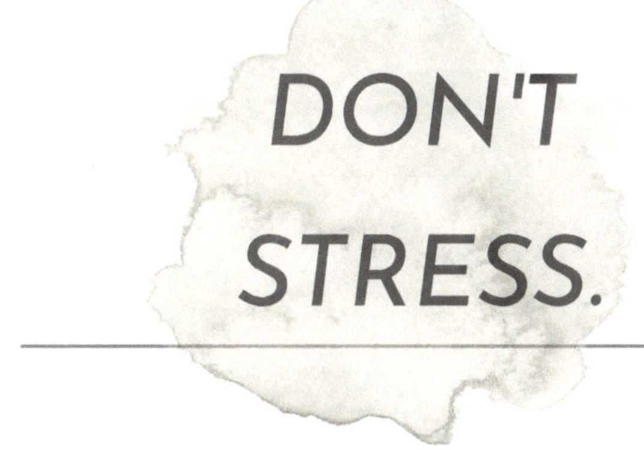

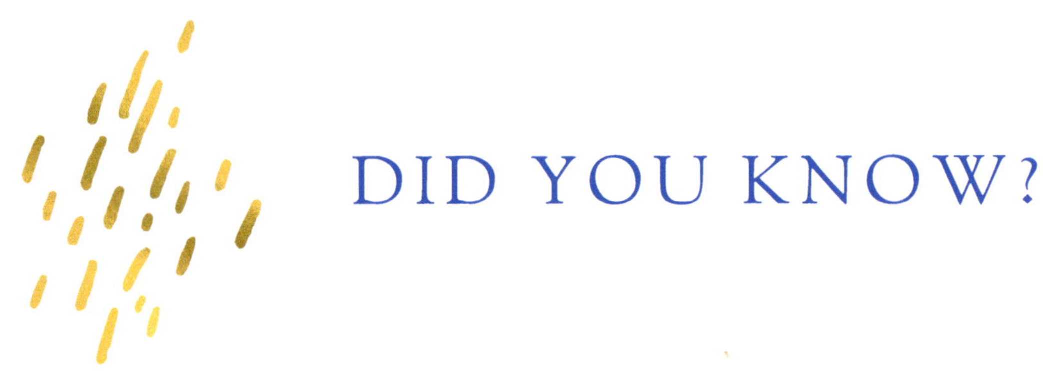

DID YOU KNOW?

What you don't know really can hurt you. High blood pressure can affect you for months or years, and one may never know it until it's too late. If you become aware, consider yourself blessed. And know that it's not silent in you any longer. At that point, it's up to you to do something about it. It can be a shocker and even overwhelming, but be grateful that you found out what is attacking you.

When I realized that I had this struggle living on the inside that I didn't invite in, I became very frustrated. I didn't embrace the lifestyle change at first either, but I realized it wouldn't get any better unless I decided to make some changes.

The first thing that must change when you want a healthier life is your mindset. No more pity parties or crying at night. No more, "Why me?" It will help if you are determined and focused. Your mind must be willing to accept the new mindset and lifestyle changes. So, that means no pity party. No more feeling down on yourself.

The change is here, and the change must start right now! Your mind must change. Start rethinking about "A New You." What you are eating or when you are starting to workout, may worry and stress you out! Stress brings distrust factors into our lives and more illness. Picture a "New You" mind, body, and soul. So let's work on a mind game.

Set your mind on the goal that you have visualized for yourself. It will help if you focus your mind on fulfilling it with plans you want to accomplish.

I hope you want to accomplish feeling better, having more energy, and having a better life for yourself. So, the mind must be programmed and educated to see the possibilities of getting better.

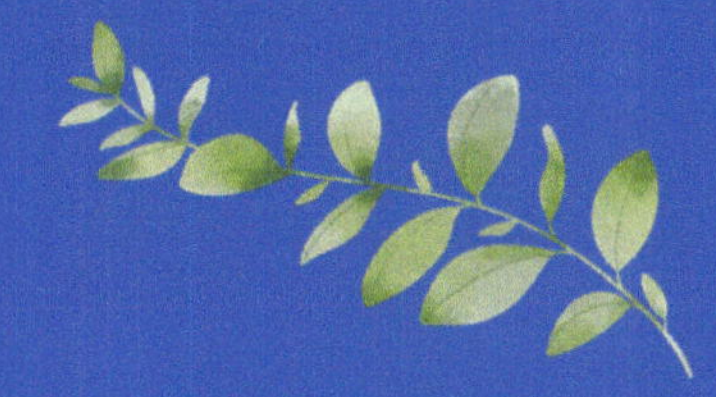

DO NOT FORGET, YOU ARE AWESOME.

EAT FOR LIFE

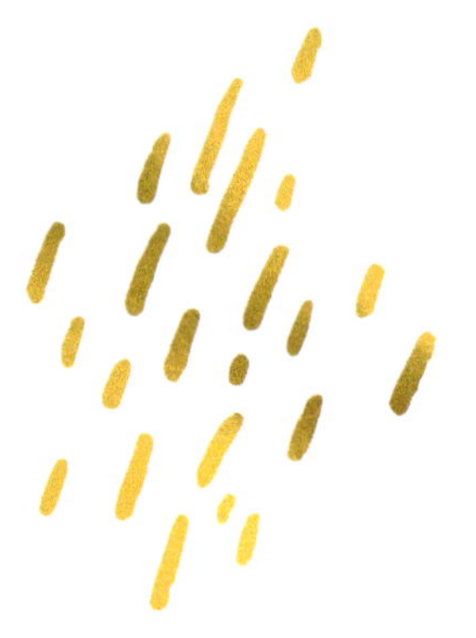

Fresh food will help boost your energy. It will also help improve your skin. Drinking lots of water helps the body stay hydrated. Eat right, snack less. Set a goal & stick to it!

What you eat matters to your body.

Reduce the amount of sugar, white flour, candy, and processed foods you consume.

Tip: Generally, if it's in a box, it's processed.

"When you start eating food without labels, you no longer need to count calories." -Amanda Kraft.

Healthy eating starts with healthy thinking.

Ask yourself:
1. Are most of my meals in a box?
2. How do I feel about eating fresh foods?
3. Do I want to have energy or not?

- **Be confident**
- **Be focused**
- **Be determined**
- **Love yourself**
- **Exercise**
- **Have a healthy mind**
- **Expect results**

LORD, GIVE ME STRENGTH IN MY PRAYER LIFE

"He who kneels before God can stand before anyone." -Unknown

Prayer is not a side thing; it's the main thing.
You've got to know that God is fighting for you!
God wants to talk to you!

If you don't know, prayer works every time.
Seek the Lord for the answer.
Wait on the Lord for direction and instructions.
Apply His plan to your life; watch God move as you obey His commands.

WRITE A PRAYER HERE ASKING GOD FOR DIRECTION AND INSTRUCTION:

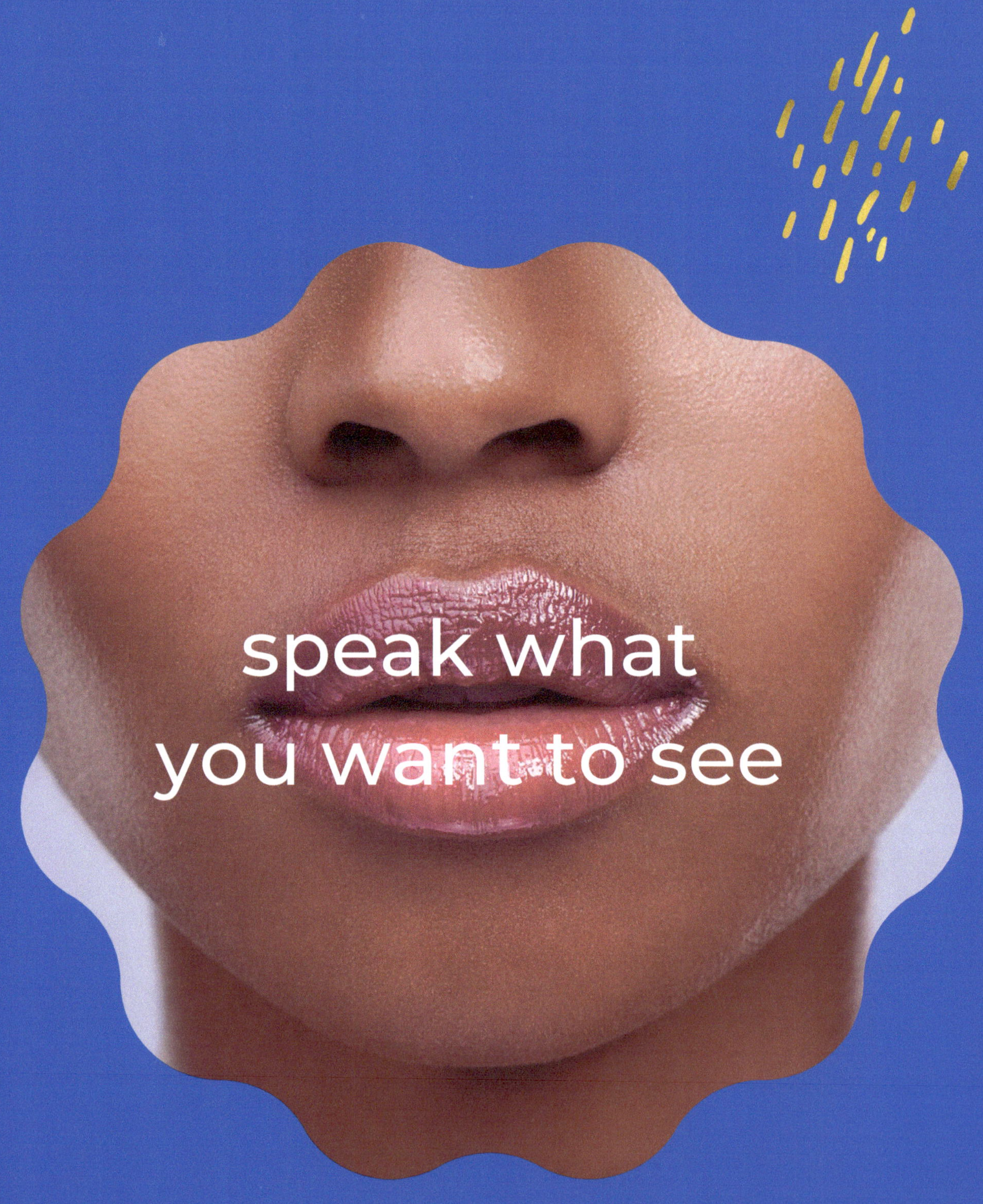

speak what
you want to see

Death and life are in the power of the tongue:
and they that love it shall eat the fruit thereof.
Proverbs 18:21

AFFIRMATIONS

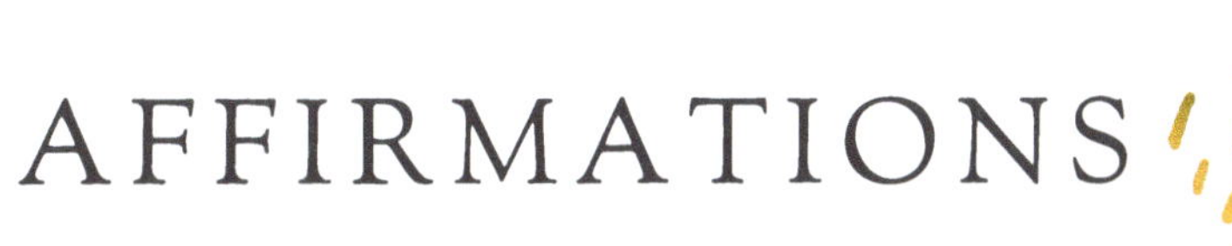

- Push yourself because the results are worth it.
- I am motivated to work on my spirit, body, and mind.
- I am determined.
- I am all that I need to be successful.
- I am confident about my health and fitness goals.
- My mind is ready, and so is my body.
- When I look in the mirror, I see muscles forming, making me happy.
- I am disciplined.
- I am transforming my body by putting it into motion every day.
- I am becoming stronger mentally as well as physically.
- I celebrate even the littlest successes.
- I am confident that I will reach my goals.
- Great results require sweat.
- Work it, and you will get it.
- I can't quit now! I have accomplished too much.
- The mirror tells no lies.
- I will exercise today no matter what.
- Working out 100% today will guarantee that you will get 100% satisfaction.
- My body looks better when I workout.
- I've got to do it no matter what!
- My best body is on the way.
- I tell myself the truth.
- Speak life, eat healthy, and workout.
- I am locked and loaded with the truth.

"Words satisfy the soul as food satisfies the stomach; the right words on a person's lip bring satisfaction." Proverbs 18:20

WHAT DOES GOD SAY ABOUT STRESS?

God does not want us to be stressed out.
He gives us principles in His Word that keeps us from being burnt out. Start with the Mind and renew your spirit, soul, and body.

Scripture to meditate and memorize:
"And without faith, it is impossible to please God because anyone who comes to him must believe that he exists and rewards those who earnestly seek him." Hebrews 11:6

How will you use faith to help you relieve stress and change your mindset?

The Mind is the beginning of change. When the mind changes everything else falls into place. Exactly, what state of mind are you in now?

LORD, I AM STRESSED OUT!

Here are some ways that STRESS can affect your body:

Head

Mood swings, anger, depression, irritability,
sadness and a lack of energy, swings in appetite,
concentration problems, sleeping issues, headaches
body aches and pain, mental health issues, and panic attacks.

Heart

Increased blood pressure, increased heartbeat
high cholesterol, instant heart attack.

Stomach

Stomach cramps, acid reflux, nausea, and weight fluctuations

Pancreas

Diabetes

Intestines

Digestive issues: irritable bowel syndrome,
diarrhea, constipation

Reproductive System

Reduced sex drive, lower sperm production (men)
increased pain during periods (for women)

Immune System

Reduced ability to battle and recover from illnesses
High Blood Pressure

Stress can destroy your body.

STRESS
THINK ABOUT THE THINGS IN YOUR LIFE THAT ARE STRESSING YOU

WHAT'S STRESSING YOU OUT? WRITING IS A FORM OF EXPRESSIVE THERAPY. IT CAN HELP YOU RELEASE STRESS. SO, WRITE ABOUT YOUR STRESSORS:

____

____

____

____

NOW, TAKE A DEEP BREATH. TAKE A MOMENT TO BREATHE IN AND BREATHE OUT. NOW, LET'S CONCENTRATE ON RELEASING THE STRESS AND GIVING IT TO THE LORD. WRITE WHAT YOU'VE RELEASED:

____

____

____

____

MATTHEW 6:25-34 "THEREFORE I TELL YOU, DO NOT WORRY ABOUT YOUR LIFE, WHAT YOU WILL EAT OR DRINK; OR ABOUT YOUR BODY, WHAT YOU WILL WEAR." WRITE ABOUT HOW YOU WILL NO LONGER WORRY:

____

____

____

____

START YOUR OWN RESEARCH ON DEVELOPING A HEALTHIER LIFE

Make a commitment to be a better you. Write a pledge to yourself. Awaken your mind to find the right way of living a better life.

____
____
____
____
____
____
____
____
____
____
____
____
____
____
____

Get motivated. Get a better diet. Get active.
Plan for success!

IS YOUR LIFE GOING IN A CIRCLE?

"SOME PEOPLE DRIVE THEMSELVES INTO A VICIOUS CYCLE. THERE IS ALWAYS A WAY OUT; A DELIGHTFUL OPENING." -TINA PANOSSIAN

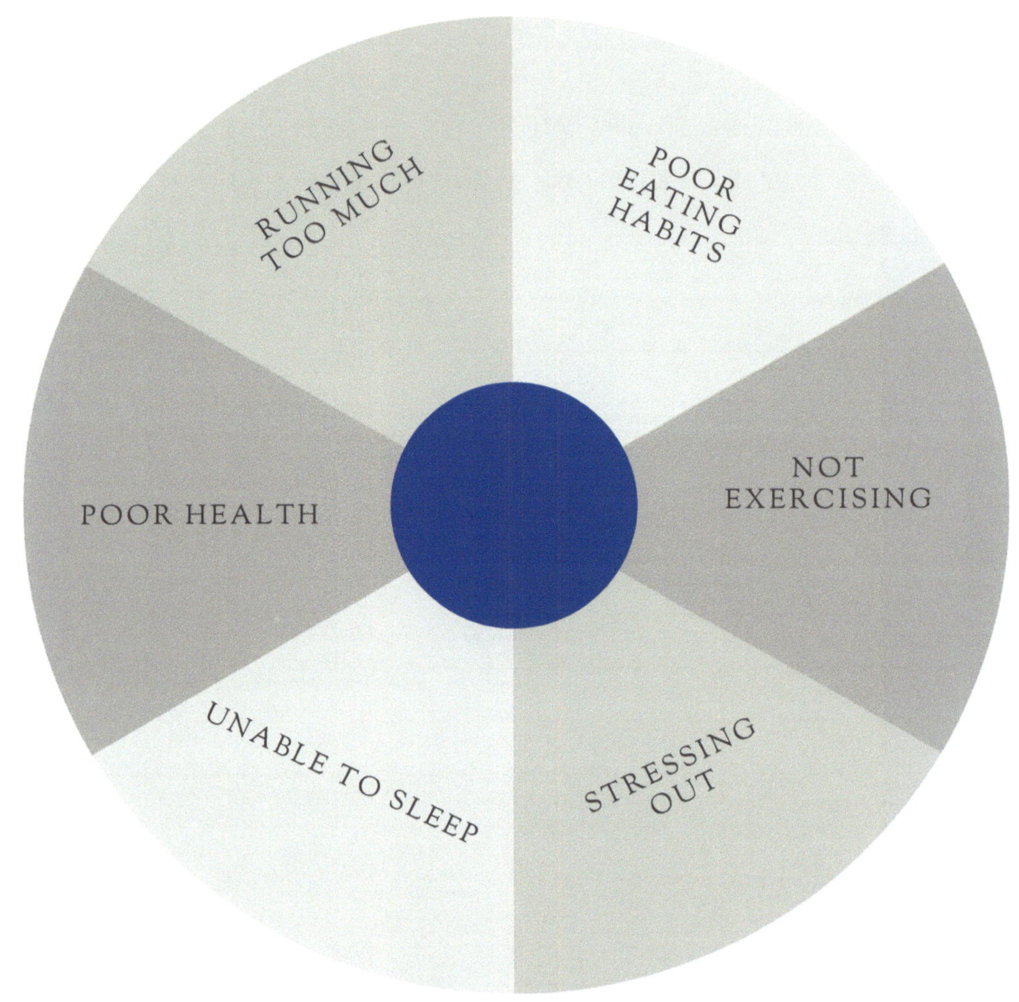

WHAT IS YOUR CIRCLE LIKE? WHAT DOES IT CONSIST OF?

GOD'S WORD CAN HEAL YOUR MIND

MEDITATE ON HIS WORD DAY AND NIGHT

Our world is filled with individuals who have troubled minds. The Word of God will heal a troubled mind. Read these scriptures and begin to apply them to your life.

John 14:27

"Peace I leave with you; my peace I give you. I do not give to you as the world gives. Do not let your hearts be troubled and do not be afraid."

Isaiah 40:29

"He gives strength to the weary and increases the power of the weak."

Luke 10:27

"And he answered, 'You shall love the Lord your God with all your heart and with all your soul and with all your strength and with all your mind, and your neighbor as yourself.'"

Romans 12:2

"Do not be conformed to this world, but be transformed by the renewal of your mind, that by testing you may discern what is the will of God, what is good and acceptable and perfect."

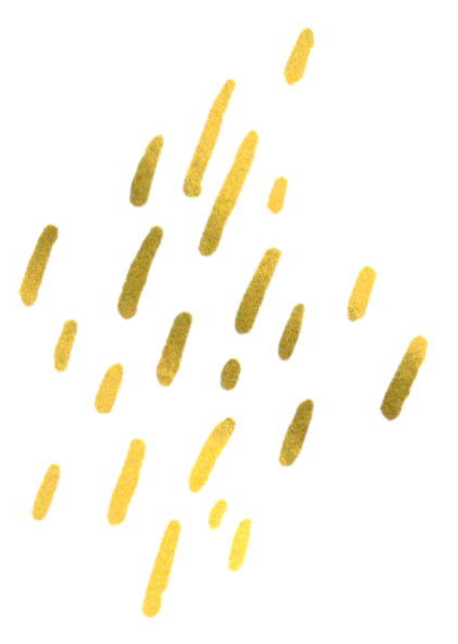

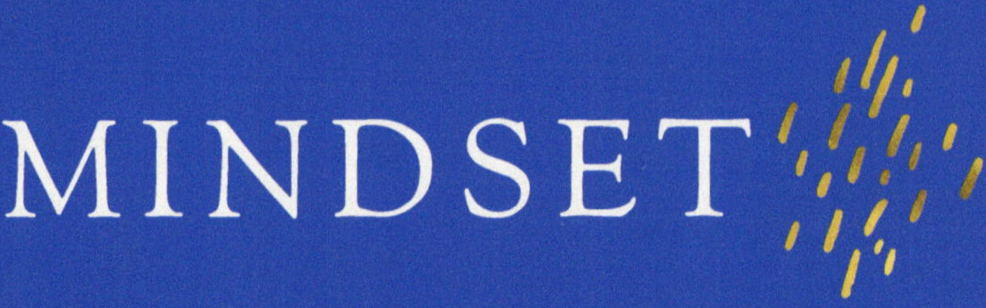

Take a deep breath, and don't panic during the pandemic.

Let's work on renewing your mind.

How can I renew my mind?

When renewing your mind, you must start by setting goals. Having the right attitude will help you see things better. Setting goals is just the beginning. You then have to formulate a plan to get there, but it happens one step at a time.

Tip: When you set a goal think positive, and stick to it.
Start by thinking positive! I use affirmations and the Word of God to start on a new path.

Scripture: "Finally, brothers and sisters, whatever is true, whatever is noble, whatever is right, whatever is pure, whatever is lovely, whatever is admirable--if anything is excellent or praiseworthy--think about such things." Philippians 4:8

WRITE SOME GOALS HERE THAT WILL HELP YOU TO RENEW YOUR MIND:

Read It: **3 John 1:2**

"Beloved, I wish above all things that thou mayest prosper and be in health, even as thy soul prospereth."

Write It:

Pray about it:

"The only way to avoid criticism: do nothing, say nothing, and be nothing." Aristotle

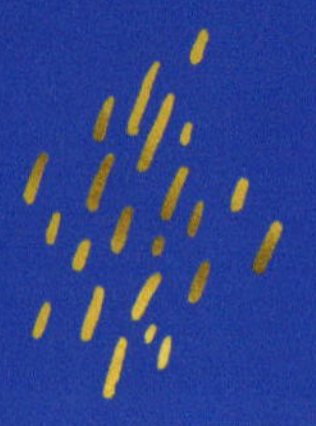

Read It: **Romans 12:1**

"Therefore I urge you, brothers and sisters, by the mercies of God, to present your bodies as a living and holy sacrifice, acceptable to God, which is your spiritual service of worship."

Write It:

Pray about it:

"The most common way people give up their power is by thinking they don't have any."
Alice Walker

Read It: **Jeremiah 33:6 King James Version**

"Behold, I will bring it health and cure, and I will cure them, and will reveal unto them the abundance of peace and truth."

Write It:

Pray about it:

"The question isn't who is going to let me; it's who is going to stop me." Ayn Rand

Read It: **Romans 12:1**

Therefore I urge you, brothers and sisters, by the mercies of God, to present your bodies as a living and holy sacrifice, acceptable to God, which is your spiritual service of worship."

Write It:

Pray about it:

"We are really competing against ourselves, we have no control over how other people perform." Pete Mashable`

"FIND OUT WHAT'S WRONG, AND ASK GOD TO SHOW YOU HOW TO FIX IT."

- COACH LILLIE

For I know the plans I have for you," declares the Lord, "plans to prosper you and not to harm you, plans to give you hope and a future.

Jeremiah 29:11

WHAT YOU WILL NEED TO START

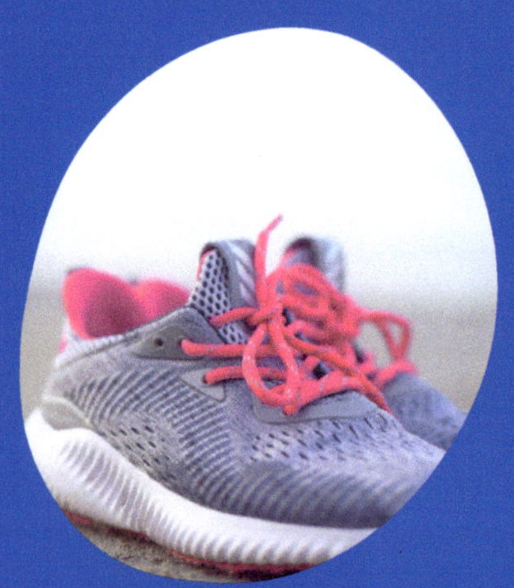

A good pair of sneakers
Playlist of upbeat praise music
1 - 64-oz. refillable water bottle
A workout partner
Your phone
Water Bottle

Exercise Benefits:
Walking is a great time for praying and communing with God.
Walking is a great time to review your Scripture memory verses.
You will have increased energy to go about your daily tasks.
You'll save lots of time getting dressed because you feel good,
your clothes fit, and you look great.

Go for a bike ride.

Get Your Body Moving. You will feel better.
Stretch for 20 minutes.
Walk for 20 minutes.

Scripture to memorize:
"She sets about her work vigorously; her arms are strong for her tasks."– Proverbs 31:17

ENGAGE

Once you engage in these things, change will come. Be determined!
A person who never gives up won't be stopped.

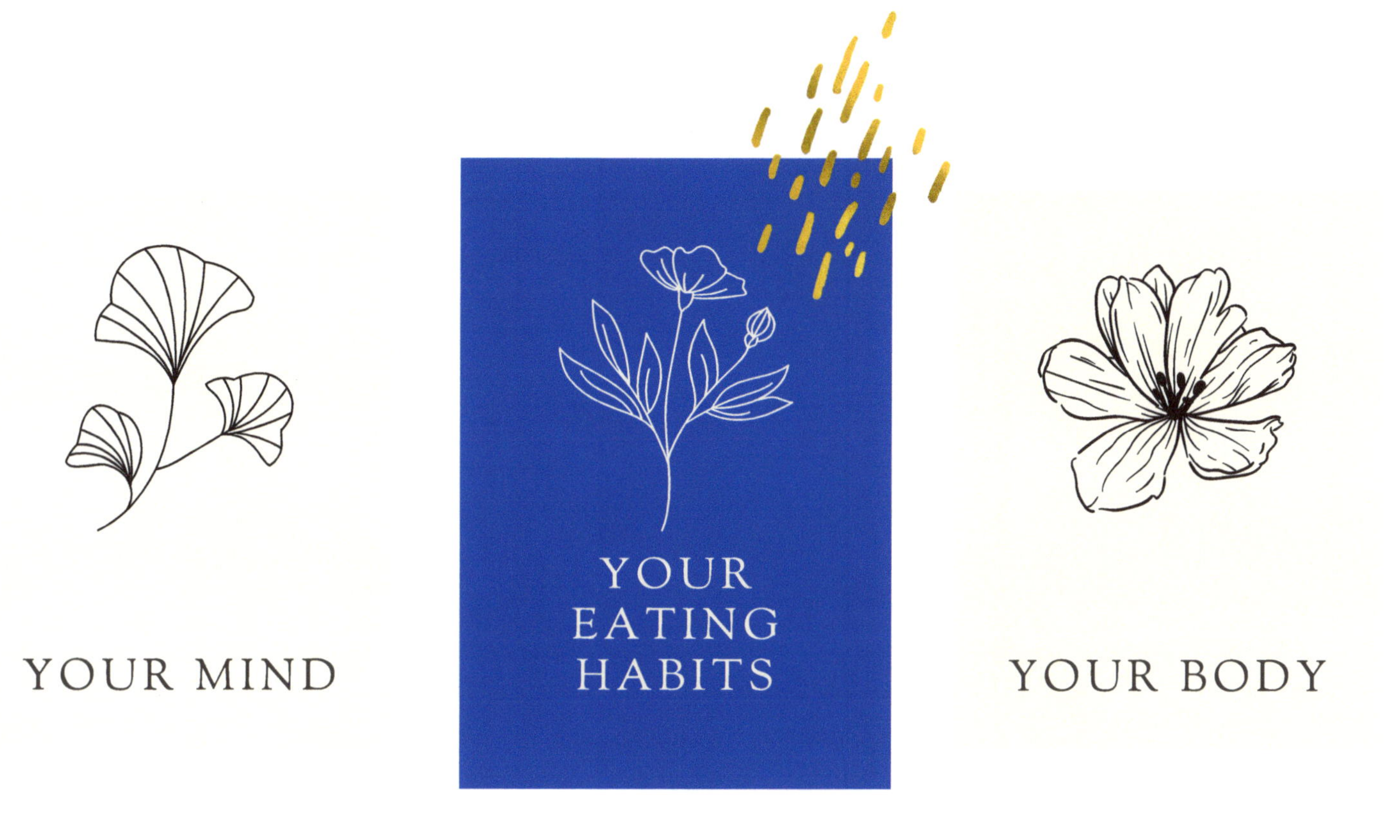

How do you plan to engage in these 3 areas?

HOW IS GOD TELLING YOU TO GET IN SHAPE?

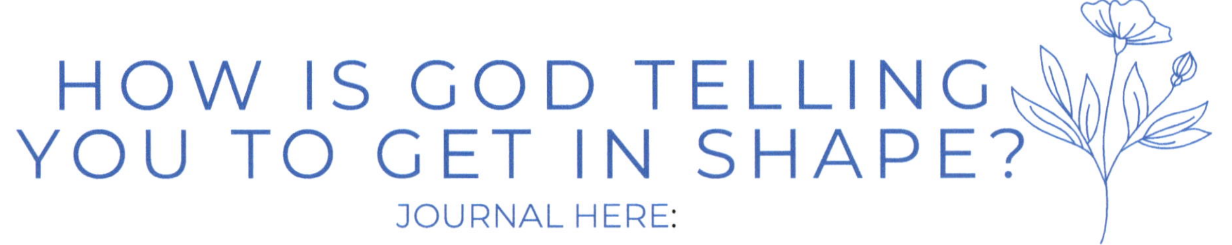

SCRIPTURE:

Name: Lillie Franks | DOB: 2/21/1964 | MRN: 108507697 | PCP: Tracy W Norfleet, MD

Diabetes

Diabetes ■

Test Results

These are your diabetes related test result components. You may view a list of all your test results for more information.

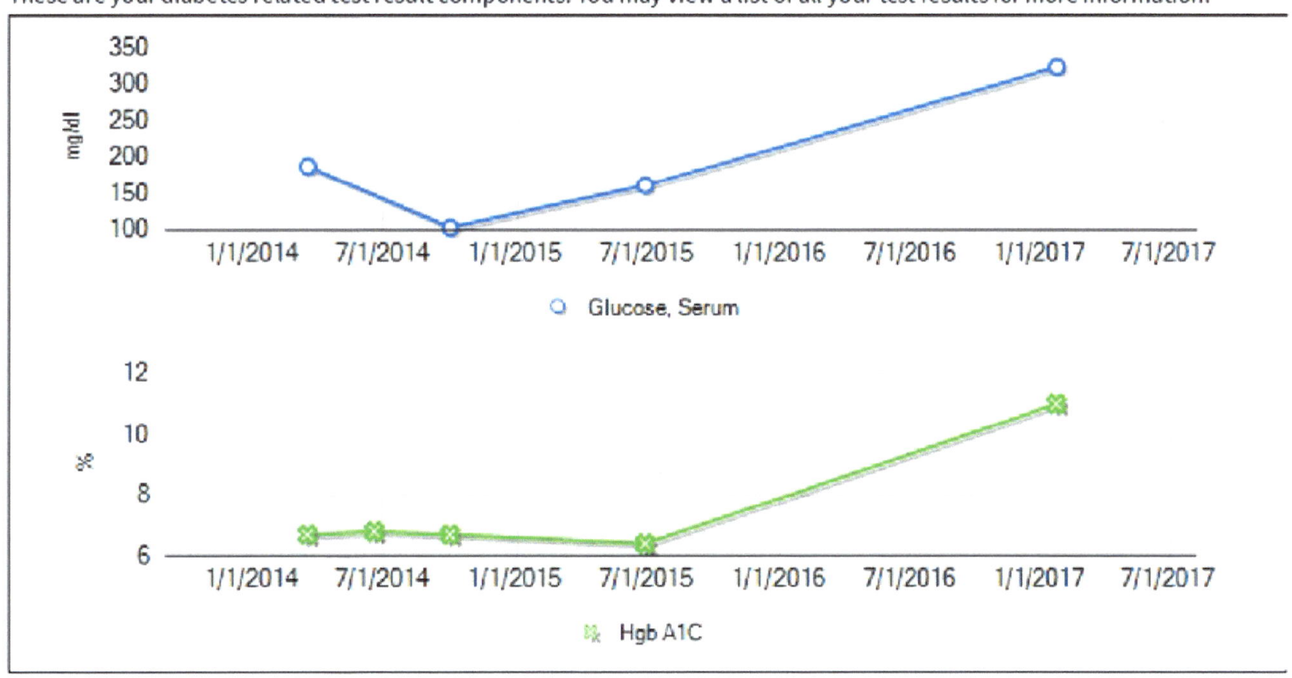

Name Standard Range	3/19/14	3/19/14	6/19/14	10/1/14	10/1/14	6/29/15	6/29/15	1/25/17	1/25/:
Glucose, Serum 70 - 199 mg/dl	187			103		161		323 H	
Hgb A1C 4.0 - 6.0 %		6.7 H	6.8 H		6.7 H		6.4 H		11.0 H

AND THE LEAVES OF THE TREE ARE FOR THE HEALING OF THE NATIONS

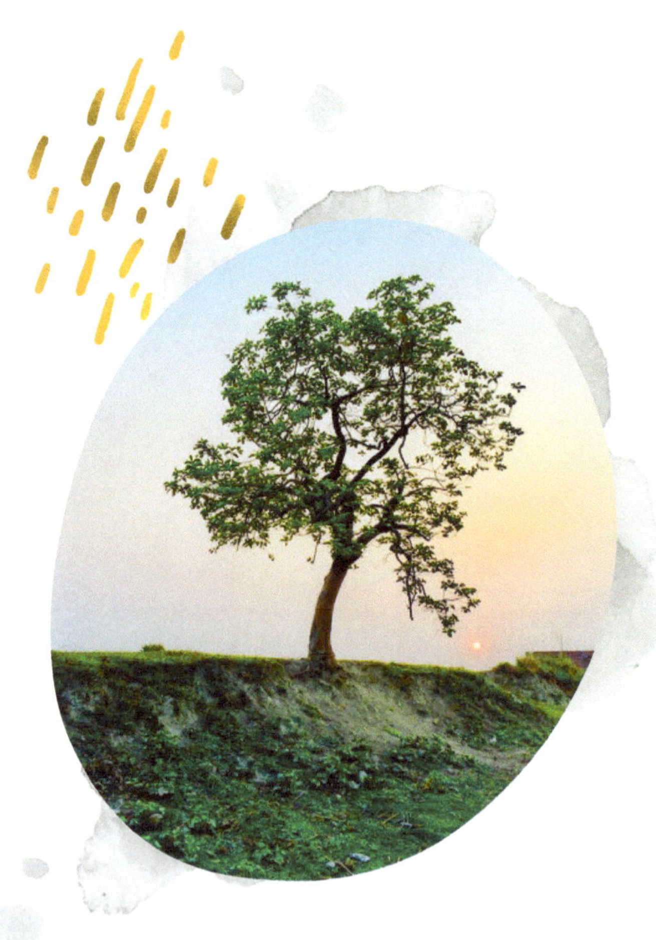

WHAT THE WORD OF GOD SAYS ABOUT HEALING LEAVES?

Revelation 22:2

"Down the middle of the great street of the city. On each side of the river stood the tree of life, bearing twelve crops of fruit, yielding its fruit every month. And the leaves of the tree are for the healing of the nations."

Ezekiel 47:12

"Fruit trees of all kinds will grow on both banks of the river. Their leaves will not wither, nor will their fruit fail. Every month they will bear fruit, because the water from the sanctuary flows to them. Their fruit will serve for food and their leaves for healing."

10 TEAS WITH HEALING BENEFITS

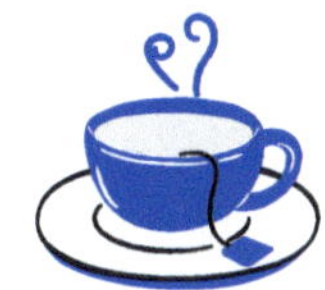

Green Tea
Treats bloating, allergies, acne and promotes weight loss

Chamomile
Great aid for sleep, relieves headaches, anxiety, bloating

Peppermint
Remedy for bloating, nausea, PMS, bad breath

Hibiscus
Helps with blood pressure, respiratory disease

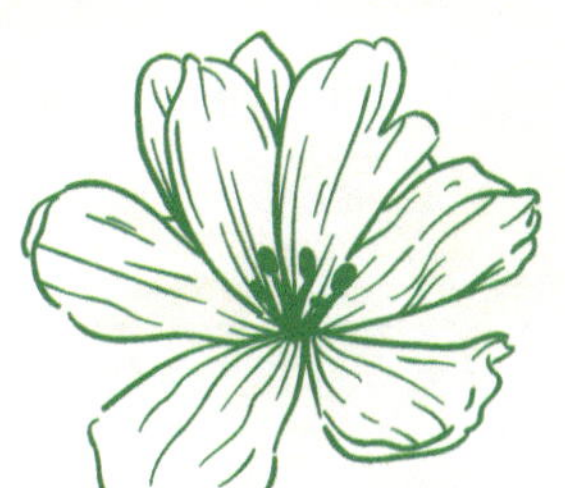

Echinacea Tea
Helps boost the immune system, which helps the body fight off viruses or infections

Black Tea
Treats anxiety, weight loss, headaches

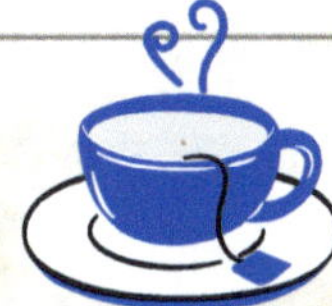

Chai Tea
Enhances immune system, fights inflammation, and cold

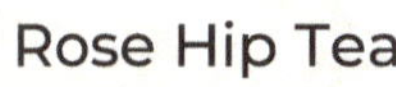

Rose Hip Tea
Reduce inflammation in people with rheumatoid arthritis and osteoarthritis.

Ginger Tea
Reduces bloating, cold, upset stomach, and sore throat

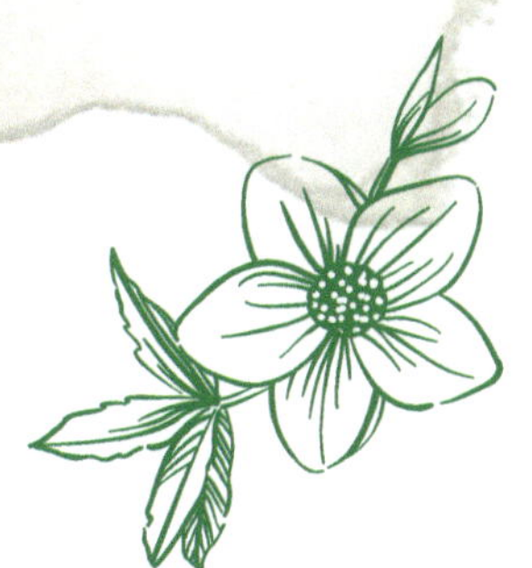

Passionflower Tea
Relieves anxiety and improves sleep

A Winner's Attitude
Perseverance, Determination, Resilience, and Confidence

STRONG MIND
"We must trust as if it all depended on God
and work as if it all depended on us."
-C. H. Spurgeon.

"Our minds have been endowed with
an incredible ability to affect the
functioning and overall health of our bodies."
-Dr. Kenneth Cooper

YOU WILL NOT BE DEFEATED

"I press on toward the goal to win the prize for which
God has called me heavenward in Christ Jesus."
Philippians 3:14

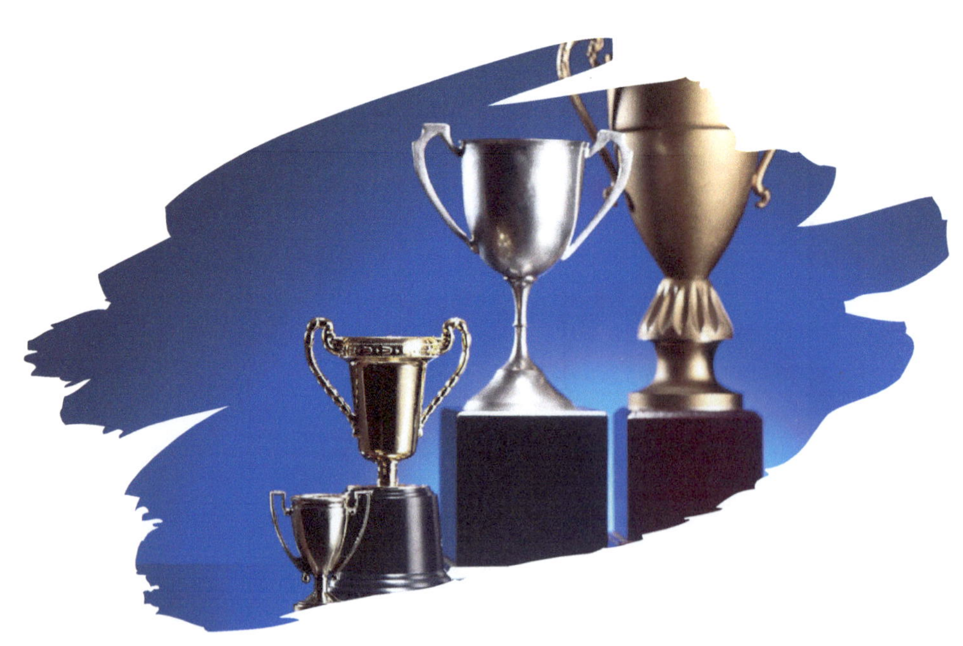

I'M GOING TO GET MY BODY BACK

SETTING GOALS AND MAKING PLANS
"I KNOW THE PLANS I HAVE YOU..." JER. 29:11

WEEK 1:

MONDAY:

TUESDAY:

WEDNESDAY:

THURSDAY:

FRIDAY:

SATURDAY:

SUNDAY:

DATE:______________________

GOALS:

____
____
____
____
____

TO DO:

____
____
____
____
____
____
____
____
____

NOTES:

____
____
____
____
____

IT'S ALL IN THE MIND

"And the peace of God, which transcends all understanding, will guard your hearts and your minds in Christ Jesus." **Phil. 4: 7**

WEEK 2:

MONDAY:

TUESDAY:

WEDNESDAY:

THURSDAY:

FRIDAY:

SATURDAY:

SUNDAY:

DATE:_______________________

GOALS:

____
____
____
____
____

TO DO:

____
____
____
____
____
____
____
____

NOTES:

____
____
____
____
____

HOW TO REVERSE THE CURSE

Beloved, I pray that all may go well with you and that you may be in good health, as it goes well with your soul." 3 John 1:2 (ESV)

WEEK 3:

MONDAY:

TUESDAY:

WEDNESDAY:

THURSDAY:

FRIDAY:

SATURDAY:

SUNDAY:

DATE:_______________________

GOALS:

____
____
____
____
____

TO DO:

____
____
____
____
____
____
____
____

NOTES:

____
____
____
____
____

WHAT'S EATING YOU?

SETTING GOALS AND MAKING PLANS

"Keep thy heart with all diligence; for out of it are the issues of life."

Proverbs 4:23 ESV

WEEK 4:

MONDAY:

TUESDAY:

WEDNESDAY:

THURSDAY:

FRIDAY:

SATURDAY:

SUNDAY:

DATE:______________________

GOALS:

TO DO:

NOTES:

I FEEL MUCH BETTER NOW!

SETTING GOALS AND MAKING PLANS

"FOR GOD GAVE US A SPIRIT NOT OF FEAR BUT OF POWER AND LOVE AND SELF-CONTROL" **2 TIM. 1: 7 (ESV)**

WEEK 5:

MONDAY:

TUESDAY:

WEDNESDAY:

THURSDAY:

FRIDAY:

SATURDAY:

SUNDAY:

DATE:_________________

GOALS:

____
____
____
____
____

TO DO:

____
____
____
____
____
____
____
____

NOTES:

____
____
____
____
____

HOW IS GOD TELLING YOU TO GET IN SHAPE?

YOU DID IT! YOU'VE MADE THIS 5-WEEK JOURNEY. NOW, TAKE A MOMENT AND REFLECT ON YOUR ACCOMPLISHMENTS.

"Whether you think you can or you think you can't, you're right."
~Henry Ford

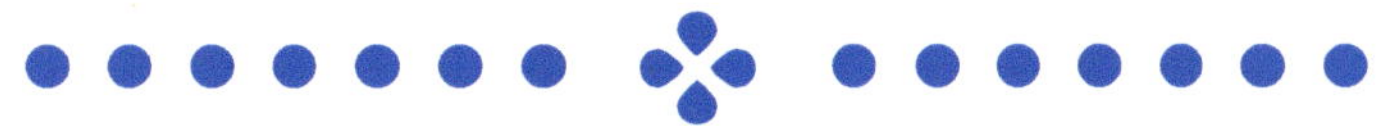

CERTIFICATE OF COMPLETION
YOU MADE IT!
YOU ARE A WINNER

THANK YOU SO MUCH FOR COMPLETING THIS JOURNEY WITH ME. I BELIEVE THAT THERE ARE GREAT THINGS IN STORE FOR THE "NEW YOU." TO MAKE IT THIS FAR, YOU HAD TO BE DETERMINED TO BE HEALTHIER. KEEP PUSHING TO OBTAIN ALL OF YOUR GOALS.

TODAY, I

____

(INSERT YOUR NAME)

JUST COMPLETED A NEW CHAPTER IN MY LIFE. THIS WORKBOOK HELPED ME WORK HARD TO TO MAINTAIN MY NEW BODY, MIND, AND SPIRIT.

MY FRIEND, LOOK IN THE MIRROR AND CELEBRATE THE "NEW YOU."

I AM SO PROUD OF YOU.

SINCERELY,

Coach Lillie

REFERENCES & PUBLISHING INFO

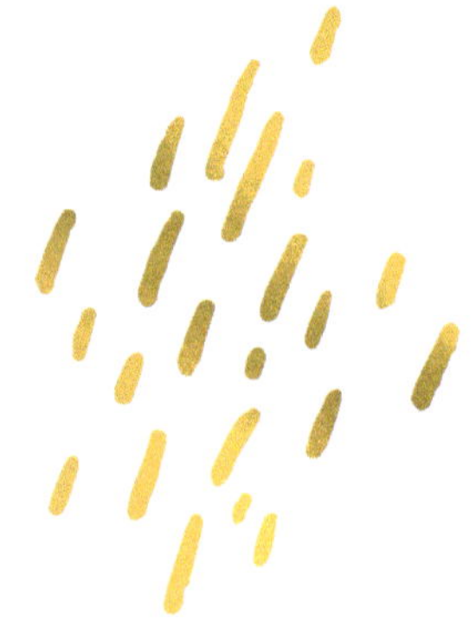

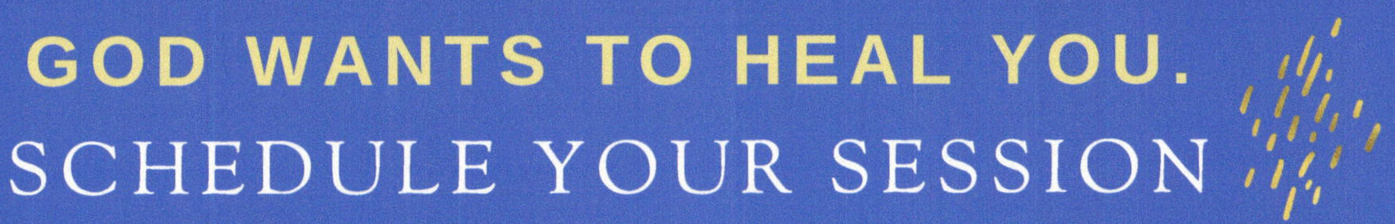

Heal me, O Lord, and I shall be healed; Save me, and I shall be saved, For You are my praise. Jeremiah 17:14

Lillie grew up with a desire to become someone impactful. She was a hard-working, dedicated student-athlete, and eventually a collegiate pageant queen (Miss Prairie View A&M, Miss Collegiate Black America). Her budding encounter with Christ would be the seed that changed her college world. She fell in love with a former track and field teammate and a God-fearing man named Michael Franks. After 42 years of friendship and over 33 years of marriage, their love is still going strong. They have two sons, four grandchildren and have embarked on the journey of leading and shepherding at New Salem M. B. Church in the city of Saint Louis, MO. She loves living her life for her Savior to the fullest. She is a Certified Life Coach, a published Author (Sister's In My Village), and she has a heart for mentoring women and girls. At New Salem, she leads a women's empowerment group once a month called Sister Circle STL. She and Pastor Franks facilitate a weekly bible for New Salem. They also conduct marriage seminars and premarital coaching sessions for couples.

God has helped her to blossom through the years. It's been challenging to get her body back after being ill and after being in a terrible accident; however, she is determined to get her body back. Tenacity, God's strength, determination, and perseverance help her to get stronger every day.

LILLIE AND MICHAEL FRANKS

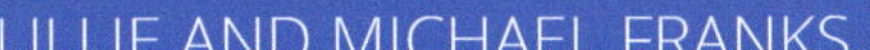

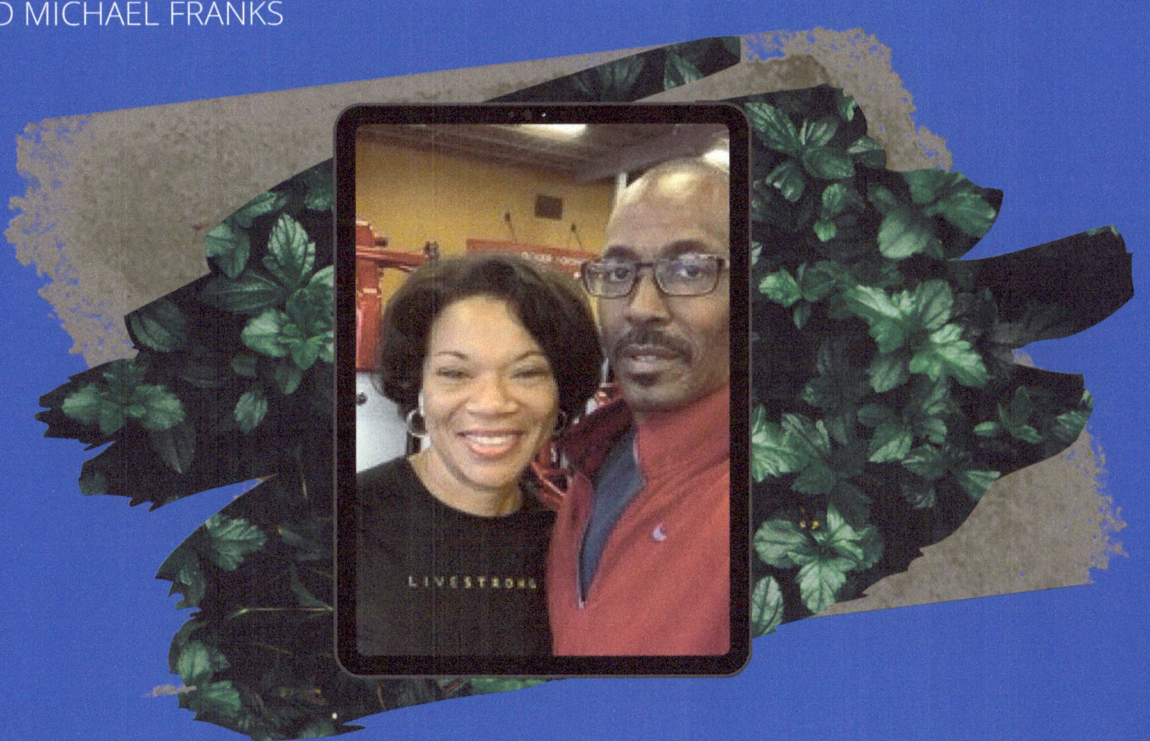

www.ingramcontent.com/pod-product-compliance
Lightning Source LLC
Chambersburg PA
CBHW040145240726
48664CB00002B/599